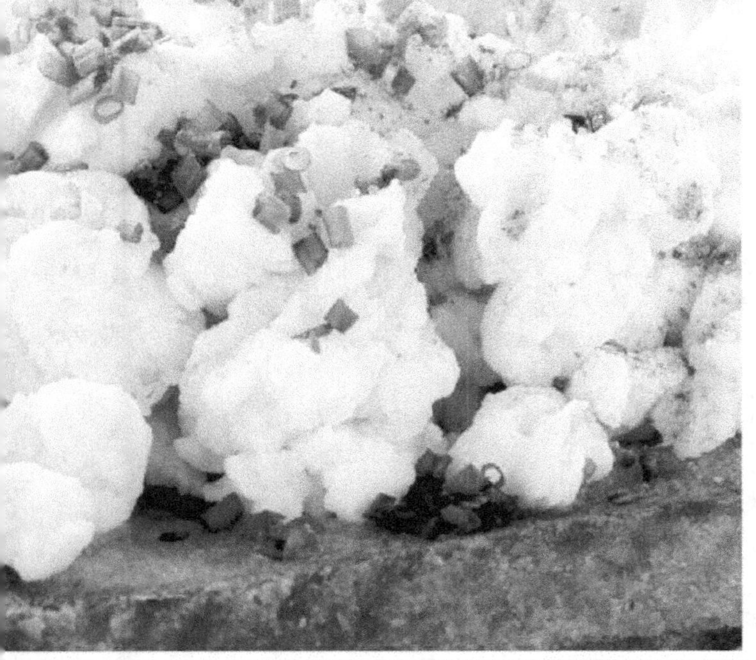

HEALTHY
Breakfast
RECIPES

CARI HENDRIX

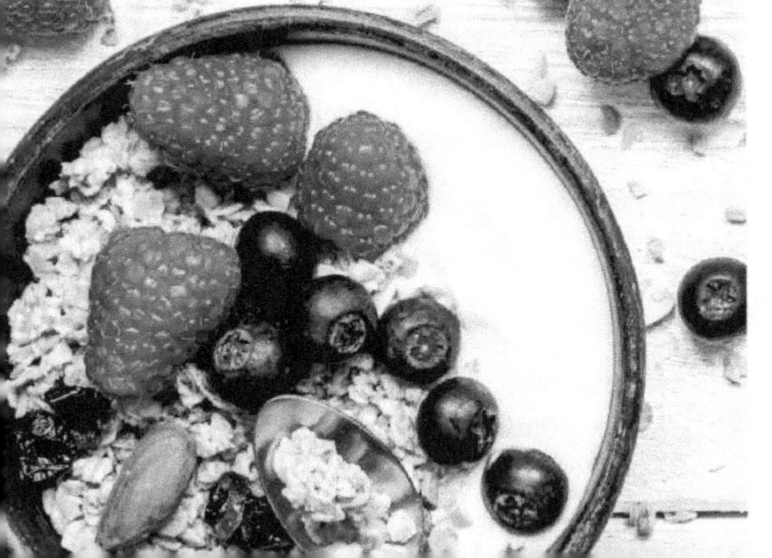
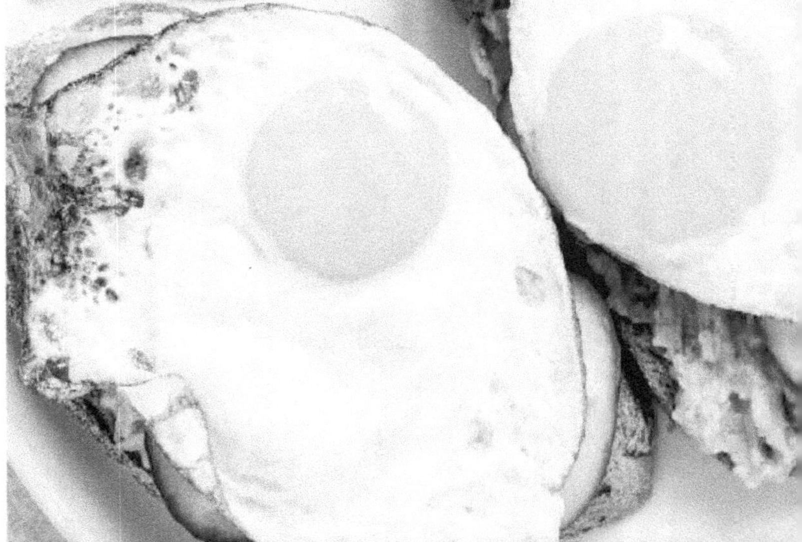

Healthy Breakfast Recipes

Welcome!

This cookbook is dedicated to helping you kickstart your day with nutritious and delicious breakfast options. A healthy breakfast is the foundation of a productive day, providing you with the energy and nutrients needed to fuel both your body and mind. In this cookbook, you'll find a variety of mouthwatering recipes that cater to different tastes and dietary preferences, from savory to sweet and everything in between. Whether you're a busy professional, a student, or just looking to make healthier choices, these recipes will inspire you to create a satisfying breakfast that promotes well-being and vitality.

Table Of Contents

Table Of Contents

Smoothie Sensations

<u>Banana-Berry Blast</u>

Ingredients:

1 ripe banana

1/2 cup of mixed berries (strawberries, blueberries, raspberries)

1/2 cup of Greek yogurt 1/2 cup of almond milk (or any milk of your choice)

1 tablespoon of honey or maple syrup (optional, for sweetness)

1/2 cup of ice cubes (optional, for thickness)

Instructions:

Peel the ripe banana and place it in a blender.

Add the mixed berries to the blender.

Spoon in the Greek yogurt.

Pour in the almond milk.

Adjust the amount to achieve your desired smoothie consistency;

add more for a thinner smoothie or less for a thicker one.

If you prefer a sweeter smoothie, add honey or maple syrup to taste.

For a colder and thicker smoothie, toss in some ice cubes.

Blend everything on high until the mixture is smooth and creamy, usually

for about 30 seconds to 1 minute.

Taste the smoothie and adjust the sweetness or thickness as needed by

adding more honey, milk, or ice.

Pour your Banana-Berry Blast into a glass, garnish with a few fresh berries or

a banana slice, if desired, and enjoy!

<u>Green Power Smoothie</u>

Ingredients:

1 cup of spinach leaves (fresh or frozen)
1/2 ripe avocado
1/2 banana
1/2 cup of pineapple chunks (fresh or frozen)
1/2 cup of coconut water
1/2 cup of plain Greek yogurt
1 tablespoon of honey or agave nectar (optional, for sweetness)
Ice cubes (optional)

Instructions:

Wash the spinach leaves thoroughly if using fresh spinach.
Cut the avocado in half, remove the pit, and scoop out the flesh.
Place the spinach, avocado, banana, pineapple chunks, Greek yogurt, and coconut water in a blender.

If you prefer a sweeter smoothie, add honey or agave nectar to taste.
Add ice cubes if you want a colder and thicker smoothie.
Blend all the ingredients on high until the smoothie is creamy and well combined, which should take about 1-2 minutes.

Taste the smoothie and adjust the sweetness or thickness as needed.
Pour your Green Power Smoothie into a glass, and it's ready to enjoy!
Feel free to adjust the ingredients and quantities to suit your taste preferences and dietary requirements.

<u>Peanut Butter & Chocolate Protein Shake</u>

Ingredients:

1 ripe banana
2 tablespoons of natural peanut butter
1 tablespoon of unsweetened cocoa powder
1 cup of unsweetened almond milk (or any milk you prefer)
1 scoop of chocolate protein powder
1/2 teaspoon of vanilla extract
1/2 cup of ice cubes (optional)

Instructions:

Peel the banana and place it in a blender.
Add the natural peanut butter, unsweetened cocoa powder, almond milk, chocolate protein powder, and vanilla extract to the blender.

If you want a colder shake, include some ice cubes.
Blend all the ingredients on high until the shake is smooth and creamy, typically for about 1-2 minutes.

Taste the shake and adjust the sweetness or thickness by adding more almond milk or cocoa powder if necessary.

Pour your Peanut Butter & Chocolate Protein Shake into a glass, and enjoy the rich and indulgent flavors!

Tropical Paradise Smoothie Bowl

Ingredients:

1/2 cup of frozen mango chunks
1/2 cup of frozen pineapple chunks
1/2 banana
1/2 cup of coconut milk (canned or carton)
1 tablespoon of shredded coconut
1 tablespoon of chia seeds
Fresh tropical fruit slices (e.g., kiwi, papaya, or passion fruit) for topping

Instructions:

In a high-speed blender, combine the frozen mango chunks, frozen
pineapple chunks, banana, and coconut milk.
Blend on high until the mixture is smooth and creamy.
You may need to pause and scrape down the sides of the blender a few
times to ensure even blending.
Pour the tropical smoothie into a bowl.
Top the smoothie bowl with shredded coconut, chia seeds, and slices of
fresh tropical fruit.

Enjoy your Tropical Paradise Smoothie Bowl with a spoon, savoring the
refreshing flavors and tropical vibes! Feel free to get creative with toppings
and adjust the consistency by adding more or less coconut milk as needed.

Enjoy these healthy and delicious smoothie sensations as part of your
balanced breakfast routine!

Hearty Breakfast Bowls

<u>Quinoa Breakfast Bowl</u>

Ingredients:

1/2 cup quinoa (uncooked)
1 cup almond milk (or your choice of milk)
1/2 teaspoon vanilla extract
1 tablespoon honey or maple syrup (optional, for sweetness)
1/2 cup mixed berries (strawberries, blueberries, raspberries)
1/4 cup chopped nuts (e.g., almonds, walnuts, or pecans)
1 tablespoon chia seeds
Sliced banana or other fruits for topping
Greek yogurt (optional, for extra creaminess)

Instructions:

Rinse the quinoa thoroughly under cold water.
In a saucepan, combine the quinoa, almond milk, and vanilla extract.
Bring it to a boil over medium heat.
Reduce the heat to low, cover, and simmer for about 15-20 minutes, or until the quinoa is cooked and has absorbed most of the liquid.
Stir occasionally. If desired, sweeten the cooked quinoa with honey or maple syrup.
Divide the cooked quinoa into serving bowls.
Top each bowl with mixed berries, chopped nuts, chia seeds, and sliced banana or other fruits.

Optionally, add a dollop of Greek yogurt for extra creaminess.

Serve your Quinoa Breakfast Bowl warm and enjoy the combination of textures and flavors!

<u>Greek Yogurt and Granola Parfait</u>

Ingredients:

1 cup Greek yogurt (plain or flavored)
1/2 cup granola 1/2 cup mixed berries (strawberries, blueberries, raspberries)
1 tablespoon honey or maple syrup (optional, for sweetness)
Sliced banana or other fruits for topping
Chopped nuts (e.g., almonds or walnuts) for extra crunch (optional)

Instructions:
In a glass or bowl, start by layering half of the Greek yogurt.
Add half of the granola on top of the yogurt layer.

Drizzle honey or maple syrup over the granola for sweetness, if desired. Layer half of the mixed berries and some sliced banana or other fruits over the granola.
Repeat the layers with the remaining yogurt, granola, mixed berries, and fruits.

Finish with a sprinkle of chopped nuts if you like an extra crunch.

Serve your Greek Yogurt and Granola Parfait immediately for a delightful and satisfying breakfast.

<u>Acai Bowl with Fresh Fruit</u>

Ingredients:

2 packets of frozen acai puree (unsweetened)
1/2 cup frozen mixed berries
1/2 banana
1/2 cup almond milk (or your choice of milk)
1 tablespoon honey or maple syrup (optional, for sweetness)
Fresh fruit slices (e.g., banana, strawberries, kiwi)
Granola for topping
Chia seeds or shredded coconut for garnish (optional)

Instructions:

Run the frozen acai packets under warm water for a few seconds to slightly
thaw them.
In a blender, combine the thawed acai puree, frozen mixed berries, banana,
almond milk, and honey or maple syrup (if desired).
Blend on high until the mixture is smooth and creamy.
Pour the acai smoothie into a bowl.

Top the acai bowl with fresh fruit slices, granola, and, if you like, a sprinkle of
chia seeds or shredded coconut for extra texture and flavor.

Enjoy your Acai Bowl with Fresh Fruit immediately as a refreshing and
nutrient-packed breakfast!

<u>Savory Oatmeal Bowl</u>

Ingredients:

1/2 cup rolled oats
1 cup water or vegetable broth
Salt and pepper to taste
1/2 avocado, sliced Cherry tomatoes, halved
Poached or fried egg (optional)
Fresh herbs (e.g., cilantro or parsley) for garnish

Instructions:

In a saucepan, bring the water or vegetable broth to a boil.
Stir in the rolled oats and reduce the heat to a simmer.
Cook the oats, stirring occasionally, for about 5-7 minutes or until they reach your desired consistency.
Season the oats with salt and pepper to taste.
Transfer the savory oatmeal to a bowl.
Top the oatmeal with sliced avocado and cherry tomatoes.

Optionally, add a poached or fried egg for extra protein and richness.

Garnish with fresh herbs for a burst of flavor.
Serve your Savory Oatmeal Bowl hot and savor the savory goodness!

Feel free to customize these hearty breakfast bowls with your favorite ingredients and adjust the sweetness or seasoning to suit your taste.

Enjoy these nutritious and satisfying breakfast options!

Scrambles & Omelets

<u>Spinach and Feta Egg White Omelet</u>

Ingredients:

4 large egg whites 1/4 cup fresh spinach, chopped
2 tablespoons crumbled feta cheese
Salt and pepper to taste
Cooking spray or a small amount of olive oil

Instructions:

In a bowl, whisk the egg whites until they are well combined.

Season with a pinch of salt and pepper.

Heat a non-stick skillet over medium heat and lightly coat it with cooking spray or a small amount of olive oil.
Pour the whisked egg whites into the skillet.

As the egg whites start to set, sprinkle the chopped spinach and crumbled feta cheese evenly over one-half of the omelet.

Carefully fold the other half of the omelet over the spinach and feta filling. Cook for another 2-3 minutes until the omelet is fully set and the cheese is melted.

Slide the omelet onto a plate, garnish with a bit more feta if desired, and serve your Spinach and Feta Egg White Omelet while it's hot and fluffy!

<u>Veggie-Packed Breakfast Scramble</u>

Ingredients:

2 large eggs 1/4 cup bell peppers, diced (a mix of red, green, or yellow)
1/4 cup onion, diced
1/4 cup baby spinach, chopped
1/4 cup cherry tomatoes, halved Salt and pepper to taste
Cooking spray or a small amount of olive oil

Instructions:

In a bowl, whisk the eggs until the yolks and whites are well combined.
Season with a pinch of salt and pepper.
Heat a non-stick skillet over medium heat and lightly coat it with cooking
spray or a small amount of olive oil.
Add the diced bell peppers and onions to the skillet and sauté for 2-3
minutes until they start to soften.
Add the baby spinach and cherry tomatoes to the skillet and continue to
cook for another 1-2 minutes until the spinach wilts and the tomatoes soften
slightly.
Pour the whisked eggs into the skillet over the sautéed vegetables.
Stir the mixture gently with a spatula, scrambling the eggs and
incorporating the veggies as they cook.
Cook until the eggs are no longer runny but still moist, which typically takes
about 2-3 minutes.

Season with a bit more salt and pepper if needed.

Serve your Veggie-Packed Breakfast Scramble on a plate, and enjoy a
nutritious and colorful start to your day!

<u>Smoked Salmon and Avocado Scramble</u>

Ingredients:

3 large eggs
2 ounces smoked salmon, chopped
1/4 ripe avocado, diced
1 tablespoon fresh chives, chopped
Salt and pepper to taste
Cooking spray or a small amount of olive oil

Instructions:

In a bowl, whisk the eggs until the yolks and whites are well combined.

Season with a pinch of salt and pepper.

Heat a non-stick skillet over medium heat and lightly coat it with cooking spray or a small amount of olive oil.

Pour the whisked eggs into the skillet.

As the eggs start to set, add the chopped smoked salmon, diced avocado, and fresh chives evenly across the eggs.

Gently stir the mixture with a spatula, continuing to cook until the eggs are fully scrambled and the salmon is heated through, which usually takes about 2-3 minutes.

Season with a bit more salt and pepper if desired.

Transfer your Smoked Salmon and Avocado Scramble to a plate, garnish with extra chives, if you like, and enjoy this luxurious and protein-packed breakfast!

<u>Vegan Tofu Scramble</u>

Ingredients:

1/2 block of extra-firm tofu, crumbled
1/4 cup bell peppers, diced
1/4 cup onion, diced
1/4 cup baby spinach, chopped
1/4 cup cherry tomatoes, halved
1/2 teaspoon turmeric powder (for color)
1/2 teaspoon garlic powder
Salt and pepper to taste
Cooking spray or a small amount of olive oil

Instructions:

Heat a non-stick skillet over medium heat and lightly coat it with cooking
spray or a small amount of olive oil.
Add the diced bell peppers and onions to the skillet and sauté for 2-3
minutes until they start to soften.
Crumble the extra-firm tofu into the skillet with the sautéed veggies.
Stir in the turmeric powder, garlic powder, salt, and pepper.
The turmeric provides a vibrant yellow color to mimic scrambled eggs.
Cook the tofu scramble for 4-5 minutes, stirring occasionally, until it's heated
through and slightly crispy.
Add the baby spinach and cherry tomatoes to the skillet and cook for
another 1-2 minutes until the spinach wilts and the tomatoes soften slightly.
Taste and adjust the seasoning if needed.
Serve your Vegan Tofu Scramble on a plate and enjoy a plant-based, protein-
rich breakfast that's both delicious and satisfying!
Feel free to customize these scrambles and omelets with your favorite
veggies, herbs, or spices to create your perfect breakfast combination.

Enjoy your hearty and flavorful breakfast!

Sandwiches & Wraps

<u>Avocado and Egg Breakfast Sandwich</u>

Ingredients:

1 whole-grain English muffin or bagel, split and toasted
1 large egg 1/2 ripe avocado, sliced
1 slice of tomato
1 slice of cheese (optional)
Salt and pepper to taste
Cooking spray or a small amount of butter (for cooking the egg)

Instructions:

Heat a non-stick skillet over medium heat and lightly coat it with cooking spray or a small amount of butter.
Crack the egg into the skillet and cook it to your desired level of doneness (e.g., fried, scrambled, or poached).
Season with salt and pepper.
While the egg is cooking, slice the avocado and tomato.
Once the egg is done, assemble your breakfast sandwich.
Start with the toasted English muffin or bagel.
Place the cooked egg on one half of the muffin or bagel.
Top the egg with avocado slices, a slice of tomato, and, if desired, a slice of cheese.
Complete the sandwich with the other half of the muffin or bagel.

Serve your Avocado and Egg Breakfast Sandwich and enjoy a satisfying and nutritious breakfast!

Greek Yogurt and Berry Breakfast Wrap

Ingredients:

1 whole-grain or whole-wheat tortilla
1/2 cup Greek yogurt (plain or flavored)
1/2 cup mixed berries (strawberries, blueberries, raspberries)
1 tablespoon honey or maple syrup (optional, for sweetness)
1/4 cup granola

Instructions:

Lay the tortilla flat on a clean surface. In the center of the tortilla, spread a layer of Greek yogurt, leaving a small border around the edges. Scatter the mixed berries evenly over the yogurt.

If you prefer a sweeter wrap, drizzle honey or maple syrup over the berries.

Sprinkle granola over the top of the berries. Fold in the sides of the tortilla and then roll it up tightly, similar to a burrito.

Slice the wrap in half diagonally, if desired.

Serve your Greek Yogurt and Berry Breakfast Wrap and enjoy a delicious and portable morning meal!

<u>Smashed Chickpea Breakfast Wrap</u>

Ingredients:

1 whole-grain or whole-wheat tortilla
1/2 cup canned chickpeas, drained and rinsed
1/4 avocado, mashed
1/4 cup cherry tomatoes, halved
2 tablespoons chopped fresh cilantro or parsley
Juice of 1/2 lemon
Salt and pepper to taste

Instructions:

In a bowl, combine the chickpeas, mashed avocado, halved cherry tomatoes, chopped cilantro or parsley, and lemon juice.
Mash the chickpea mixture with a fork or potato masher until the chickpeas are partially smashed, leaving some texture.
Season the mixture with salt and pepper to taste.
Lay the tortilla flat on a clean surface.
Spread the smashed chickpea mixture evenly across the center of the tortilla.
Fold in the sides of the tortilla and then roll it up tightly, similar to a burrito.

Slice the wrap in half diagonally, if desired.

Serve your Smashed Chickpea Breakfast Wrap and savor a protein-packed and flavorful breakfast!

<u>Spinach and Mushroom Breakfast Quesadilla</u>

Ingredients:

2 whole-grain or whole-wheat tortillas
1/2 cup baby spinach leaves
1/2 cup sliced mushrooms
1/4 cup shredded cheese (e.g., cheddar or mozzarella)
2 large eggs
Salt and pepper to taste
Cooking spray or a small amount of olive oil

Instructions:

In a non-stick skillet over medium heat, sauté the sliced mushrooms until they are tender and lightly browned, about 4-5 minutes.
Remove them from the skillet and set aside.
In the same skillet, add a little cooking spray or olive oil if needed.
Crack the eggs into the skillet and cook them to your desired level of doneness (e.g., scrambled or fried).
Season with salt and pepper.
While the eggs are cooking, lay out the tortillas on a clean surface.
Divide the baby spinach leaves evenly between the two tortillas.
Sprinkle the shredded cheese over the spinach.
Once the eggs are done, divide them between the tortillas on top of the cheese.
Add the sautéed mushrooms on top of the eggs.
Fold the tortillas in half to create quesadillas.
In the same skillet, warm the quesadillas over medium heat until the cheese is melted and the tortillas are lightly toasted, about 2-3 minutes per side.

Slice the quesadillas into wedges and serve your Spinach and Mushroom Breakfast Quesadilla, enjoying the combination of flavors and textures!

Feel free to customize these breakfast sandwiches and wraps with your favorite ingredients and adjust the seasonings to suit your taste preferences.

Enjoy your tasty and convenient breakfast on the go!

Homemade Granola & Cereals

<u>Crunchy Maple-Almond Granola</u>

Ingredients:

3 cups old-fashioned oats
1 cup almonds, chopped
1/2 cup unsweetened shredded coconut
1/2 cup pure maple syrup 1/4 cup coconut oil, melted
1 teaspoon vanilla extract
1/2 teaspoon ground cinnamon
1/4 teaspoon salt
1/2 cup dried cranberries or your choice of dried fruits (optional)

Instructions:

Preheat your oven to 325°F (163°C).
Line a baking sheet with parchment paper.
In a large mixing bowl, combine the old-fashioned oats, chopped almonds, and unsweetened shredded coconut.
In a separate microwave-safe bowl or on the stovetop, melt the coconut oil and mix in the pure maple syrup, vanilla extract, ground cinnamon, and salt.
Pour the wet mixture over the dry ingredients in the large bowl and stir well until everything is evenly coated.
Spread the granola mixture evenly onto the prepared baking sheet.
Bake in the preheated oven for 20-25 minutes, or until the granola is golden brown, stirring it every 10 minutes for even cooking.
Remove the granola from the oven and let it cool completely on the baking sheet.
It will continue to crisp up as it cools. If desired, stir in the dried cranberries or your choice of dried fruits once the granola has cooled.

Store your Crunchy Maple-Almond Granola in an airtight container at room temperature.

Enjoy it with yogurt, milk, or as a topping for smoothie bowls!

<u>Overnight Oats with Chia Seeds</u>

Ingredients:

1/2 cup rolled oats
1 cup almond milk (or your choice of milk)
2 tablespoons chia seeds
1 tablespoon honey or maple syrup (optional, for sweetness)
1/2 teaspoon vanilla extract
Fresh berries or sliced fruits for topping
Nuts or seeds for garnish (e.g., sliced almonds or pumpkin seeds)

Instructions:

In a jar or container with a lid, combine the rolled oats, almond milk, chia
seeds, honey or maple syrup (if desired), and vanilla extract.
Stir the mixture until everything is well combined.

Seal the jar or container with the lid and refrigerate it overnight or for at least
4-6 hours.

This allows the oats and chia seeds to absorb the liquid and thicken.
Before serving, give the overnight oats a good stir to make sure all
ingredients are evenly distributed.

Top the oats with fresh berries or sliced fruits and a sprinkle of nuts or seeds
for added texture and flavor.

Enjoy your Overnight Oats with Chia Seeds as a nutritious and convenient
breakfast!

<u>Cinnamon-Apple Quinoa Porridge</u>

Ingredients:

1/2 cup quinoa, rinsed
1 cup water
1 cup almond milk (or your choice of milk)
1 apple, peeled, cored, and diced
1/2 teaspoon ground cinnamon
1 tablespoon honey or maple syrup (optional, for sweetness)
Chopped nuts or dried fruits for topping (optional)

Instructions:

In a saucepan, combine the rinsed quinoa, water, and almond milk.
Bring the mixture to a boil, then reduce the heat to low, cover, and simmer
for about 15-20 minutes or until the quinoa is cooked and has absorbed most
of the liquid.

While the quinoa is cooking, sauté the diced apple in a separate skillet over
medium heat with a pinch of cinnamon until it becomes tender and slightly
caramelized, about 5-7 minutes.

You can add a bit of honey or maple syrup for extra sweetness if desired.

Once the quinoa is cooked, stir in the sautéed apple and remaining ground
cinnamon.
Add honey or maple syrup for sweetness if needed.
Top your Cinnamon-Apple Quinoa Porridge with chopped nuts or dried fruits
for added texture and flavor.

Serve your warm and comforting quinoa porridge for a hearty and satisfying
breakfast!

<u>Coconut and Mixed Berry Muesli</u>

Ingredients:

1 cup rolled oats
1/2 cup unsweetened shredded coconut
1/2 cup mixed berries (strawberries, blueberries, raspberries)
1/4 cup chopped nuts (e.g., almonds or walnuts) 1/4 cup dried coconut flakes
1 cup Greek yogurt (plain or flavored)
1 tablespoon honey or maple syrup (optional, for sweetness)

Instructions:

In a large mixing bowl, combine the rolled oats, unsweetened shredded coconut, mixed berries, chopped nuts, and dried coconut flakes.

If desired, sweeten the mixture with honey or maple syrup.

Serve your Coconut and Mixed Berry Muesli in a bowl with a generous dollop of Greek yogurt. Enjoy your muesli as a wholesome and customizable breakfast!
These homemade granola and cereal recipes offer a variety of flavors and textures to suit your breakfast preferences.

Feel free to customize them with your favorite ingredients and adjust the sweetness to your liking.
Enjoy your nutritious and delicious breakfast!

Pancakes & Waffles

Whole Wheat Banana Pancakes

Ingredients:

1 cup whole wheat flour 1 tablespoon sugar (optional)
1 teaspoon baking powder
1/2 teaspoon baking soda
1/4 teaspoon salt
1 ripe banana, mashed
1 cup buttermilk (or 1 cup milk mixed with 1 tablespoon lemon juice or white vinegar)
1 large egg
1 tablespoon melted butter or vegetable oil
1/2 teaspoon vanilla extract
Sliced bananas and maple syrup for topping (optional)

Instructions:

In a large mixing bowl, whisk together the whole wheat flour, sugar (if using), baking powder, baking soda, and salt.
In a separate bowl, mash the ripe banana with a fork until it's mostly smooth.
Add the buttermilk, egg, melted butter or oil, and vanilla extract to the mashed banana.
Mix until well combined.
Pour the wet ingredients into the dry ingredients and stir until just combined.
Be careful not to overmix; a few lumps are okay.
Preheat a griddle or non-stick skillet over medium heat and lightly grease it with butter or oil. Pour 1/4 cup portions of pancake batter onto the hot griddle.
Cook the pancakes until bubbles form on the surface and the edges look set, usually about 2-3 minutes.
Flip the pancakes with a spatula and cook for an additional 2-3 minutes, or until they're golden brown on both sides and cooked through.
Remove the pancakes from the griddle and keep them warm.

Serve your Whole Wheat Banana Pancakes with sliced bananas and a drizzle of maple syrup, if desired.

Enjoy your fluffy and flavorful pancakes!

<u>Blueberry Protein Pancakes</u>
Ingredients:
1 cup whole wheat flour
1/2 cup protein powder (whey or plant-based)
1 tablespoon sugar (optional)
1 teaspoon baking powder
1/2 teaspoon baking soda
1/4 teaspoon salt
1 cup buttermilk (or 1 cup milk mixed with 1 tablespoon lemon juice or white vinegar)
1 large egg
1 tablespoon melted butter or vegetable oil 1/2 teaspoon vanilla extract 1/2 cup fresh or frozen blueberries
Sliced bananas and a drizzle of honey for topping (optional)

Instructions:

In a large mixing bowl, combine the whole wheat flour, protein powder, sugar (if using), baking powder, baking soda, and salt.
In a separate bowl, whisk together the buttermilk, egg, melted butter or oil, and vanilla extract.
Pour the wet ingredients into the dry ingredients and stir until just combined.
Don't overmix; it's okay to have a few lumps.
Gently fold in the blueberries.
Preheat a griddle or non-stick skillet over medium heat and lightly grease it with butter or oil.
Pour 1/4 cup portions of pancake batter onto the hot griddle.
Cook the pancakes until bubbles form on the surface and the edges look set, usually about 2-3 minutes.
Flip the pancakes with a spatula and cook for an additional 2-3 minutes, or until they're golden brown on both sides and cooked through.
Remove the pancakes from the griddle and keep them warm.

Serve your Blueberry Protein Pancakes with sliced bananas and a drizzle of honey, if desired.

Enjoy these protein-packed and tasty pancakes!

<u>Sweet Potato Waffles</u>

Ingredients:

1 cup whole wheat flour
1 tablespoon sugar (optional)
1 teaspoon baking powder
1/2 teaspoon baking soda
1/4 teaspoon salt
1/2 teaspoon ground cinnamon
1/4 teaspoon ground nutmeg
1 cup buttermilk (or 1 cup milk mixed with 1 tablespoon lemon juice or white vinegar)
1 large egg
1/2 cup mashed sweet potato (cooked and cooled) 2 tablespoons melted butter or vegetable oil
1/2 teaspoon vanilla extract Sliced bananas and a sprinkle of chopped nuts for topping (optional)

Instructions:

In a large mixing bowl, whisk together the whole wheat flour, sugar (if using), baking powder, baking soda, salt, ground cinnamon, and ground nutmeg.
In a separate bowl, combine the buttermilk, egg, mashed sweet potato, melted butter or oil, and vanilla extract.
Mix until well combined.
Pour the wet ingredients into the dry ingredients and stir until just combined. Be careful not to overmix; a few lumps are okay.
Preheat your waffle iron according to the manufacturer's instructions and lightly grease it with non-stick spray or oil.
Pour the waffle batter onto the preheated waffle iron, using the recommended amount for your specific waffle iron.
Cook the waffles until they're golden brown and crispy, following your waffle iron's instructions.
Remove the waffles from the iron and keep them warm.

Serve your Sweet Potato Waffles with sliced bananas and a sprinkle of chopped nuts for added texture and flavor, if desired.

Enjoy these delightful and nutritious waffles!

<u>Vegan Oatmeal Pancakes</u>

Ingredients:

1 cup rolled oats
1 cup almond milk (or your choice of plant-based milk)
1 ripe banana
1 tablespoon maple syrup or agave nectar
1/2 teaspoon vanilla extract
1/2 teaspoon ground cinnamon
1/4 teaspoon salt
1 teaspoon baking powder
1/2 teaspoon baking soda
1 tablespoon apple cider vinegar
Cooking spray or a small amount of vegetable oil for greasing the skillet

Instructions:

In a blender, combine the rolled oats, almond milk, ripe banana, maple syrup or agave nectar, vanilla extract, ground cinnamon, salt, baking powder, and baking soda.
Blend until the mixture is smooth and all ingredients are well combined.
Stir in the apple cider vinegar and let the batter sit for a few minutes to allow it to thicken.
Preheat a non-stick skillet over medium heat and lightly grease it with cooking spray or a small amount of vegetable oil.
Pour 1/4 cup portions of pancake batter onto the hot skillet.
Cook the pancakes until bubbles form on the surface and the edges look set, usually about 2-3 minutes.
Flip the pancakes with a spatula and cook for an additional 2-3 minutes, or until they're golden brown on both sides and cooked through.
Remove the pancakes from the skillet and keep them warm.

Serve your Vegan Oatmeal Pancakes with your choice of toppings, such as fresh fruit, a drizzle of maple syrup, or a dollop of dairy-free yogurt.

Enjoy these wholesome and vegan-friendly pancakes!

Baked Breakfast Delights

<u>Baked Oatmeal with Apples and Cinnamon</u>

Ingredients:
2 cups old-fashioned oats
1/2 cup chopped nuts (e.g., almonds or walnuts)
1/4 cup brown sugar or maple syrup
1 teaspoon baking powder
1 1/2 teaspoons ground cinnamon
1/4 teaspoon salt
2 cups milk (dairy or non-dairy)
1 large egg
2 tablespoons melted butter or coconut oil
1 teaspoon vanilla extract
2 cups diced apples (about 2 medium-sized apples)
Additional sliced apples, nuts, and a drizzle of honey for topping (optional)

Instructions:

Preheat your oven to 350°F (175°C).
Grease a baking dish (such as an 8x8-inch or 9x9-inch square dish) or line it with parchment paper.
In a large mixing bowl, combine the old-fashioned oats, chopped nuts, brown sugar or maple syrup, baking powder, ground cinnamon, and salt.
In another bowl, whisk together the milk, egg, melted butter or coconut oil, and vanilla extract.
Pour the wet ingredients over the dry ingredients and stir until well combined.
Gently fold in the diced apples.
Pour the mixture into the prepared baking dish, spreading it out evenly.
If desired, top the oatmeal with additional sliced apples and nuts.
Bake in the preheated oven for 35-40 minutes or until the oatmeal is set and the top is golden brown.
Remove the baked oatmeal from the oven and let it cool slightly before serving.

Serve your Baked Oatmeal with Apples and Cinnamon warm, and consider drizzling honey on top for extra sweetness, if desired.

Enjoy a warm and comforting breakfast!

<u>Breakfast Casserole with Sausage and Eggs</u>

Ingredients:

1 pound breakfast sausage (pork or turkey), cooked and crumbled
6 large eggs
1 cup milk
1 teaspoon ground mustard Salt and pepper to taste
4 cups cubed bread (e.g., French bread or white bread)
1 1/2 cups shredded cheddar cheese
Chopped fresh herbs (e.g., parsley or chives) for garnish (optional)

Instructions:

Preheat your oven to 350°F (175°C).
Grease a baking dish (such as a 9x13-inch dish).
In a large mixing bowl, whisk together the eggs, milk, ground mustard, salt, and pepper.
Add the cubed bread and half of the shredded cheddar cheese to the bowl with the eggs.
Mix until the bread is well coated.
Gently stir in the cooked and crumbled breakfast sausage.
Pour the mixture into the prepared baking dish, spreading it out evenly.
Sprinkle the remaining cheddar cheese on top.
Cover the baking dish with aluminum foil.

Bake in the preheated oven for 25-30 minutes.
Remove the foil and bake for an additional 10-15 minutes, or until the casserole is set, the top is golden brown, and a toothpick inserted into the center comes out clean.

Let the Breakfast Casserole with Sausage and Eggs cool for a few minutes before serving.

Garnish with chopped fresh herbs if desired.

Serve your hearty breakfast casserole warm, and enjoy a savory and satisfying meal!

<u>Spinach and Feta Breakfast Quiche</u>

Ingredients:

1 pre-made or homemade pie crust
6 large eggs
1 cup milk (dairy or non-dairy)
Salt and pepper to taste
1 cup fresh spinach, chopped
1/2 cup crumbled feta cheese
1/4 cup diced red bell pepper
1/4 cup diced onion
Cooking spray or a small amount of olive oil

Instructions:

Preheat your oven to 375°F (190°C).
Place the pie crust in a pie dish or tart pan.
Prick the bottom with a fork.
In a bowl, whisk together the eggs and milk.
Season with salt and pepper.

In a skillet, heat a small amount of olive oil or use cooking spray over
medium heat.
Sauté the diced red bell pepper and onion until they soften, about 2-3
minutes.
Spread the sautéed vegetables evenly over the bottom of the pie crust.
Sprinkle the chopped fresh spinach over the vegetables.
Pour the egg and milk mixture over the vegetables and spinach.

Sprinkle the crumbled feta cheese on top.

Bake in the preheated oven for 35-40 minutes or until the quiche is set and
the top is lightly golden brown.
Remove the Spinach and Feta Breakfast Quiche from the oven and let it
cool for a few minutes before slicing.

Slice and serve your quiche, either warm or at room temperature.

Enjoy a flavorful and nutritious breakfast!

<u>Blueberry Baked French Toast</u>

Ingredients:

1 loaf of day-old French bread, cut into slices
1 cup fresh or frozen blueberries
6 large eggs
1 cup milk (dairy or non-dairy)
1/4 cup maple syrup
1 teaspoon vanilla extract
1/2 teaspoon ground cinnamon
Pinch of salt
Powdered sugar and extra blueberries for topping (optional)

Instructions:

Grease a 9x13-inch baking dish.
Arrange the slices of day-old French bread in the baking dish, overlapping them slightly.
Sprinkle the blueberries evenly over the bread slices.
In a bowl, whisk together the eggs, milk, maple syrup, vanilla extract, ground cinnamon, and a pinch of salt.
Pour the egg mixture evenly over the bread and blueberries, making sure all the bread is soaked.
Cover the baking dish with aluminum foil and refrigerate it for at least 4 hours or overnight.
This allows the bread to absorb the flavors.
Preheat your oven to 350°F (175°C).
Bake the Blueberry Baked French Toast, covered with foil, in the preheated oven for 30 minutes.
Remove the foil and bake for an additional 15-20 minutes, or until the top is golden brown and the French toast is cooked through.
Let the baked French toast cool slightly before serving.
Dust with powdered sugar and garnish with extra blueberries if desired.

Serve your Blueberry Baked French Toast warm and enjoy a delightful and fruity breakfast!

These baked breakfast delight recipes offer a variety of flavors and textures to suit your morning preferences.

Enjoy these hearty and delicious breakfast options!

Homemade Breakfast Bars & Bites

<u>No-Bake Peanut Butter and Chocolate Oat Bars</u>

Ingredients:

1 1/2 cups rolled oats
1/2 cup peanut butter (or almond butter for a variation)
1/3 cup honey or maple syrup
1/3 cup mini chocolate chips
1/3 cup chopped nuts (e.g., almonds or walnuts)
1/4 cup dried cranberries or raisins (optional)
1 teaspoon vanilla extract
A pinch of salt

Instructions:

In a large mixing bowl, combine the rolled oats, mini chocolate chips, chopped nuts, and dried cranberries or raisins (if using).
In a microwave-safe bowl, warm the peanut butter and honey (or maple syrup) until they're easy to stir.
This usually takes about 20-30 seconds in the microwave.
Stir the vanilla extract and a pinch of salt into the peanut butter and honey mixture.
Pour the peanut butter mixture over the dry ingredients in the large mixing bowl.
Mix everything together until the oats and other ingredients are evenly coated with the peanut butter mixture.
Line an 8x8-inch square baking pan with parchment paper, leaving some overhang on the sides for easy removal.
Press the mixture firmly into the prepared baking pan using a spatula or your hands.
Place the pan in the refrigerator and chill for at least 1-2 hours, or until the bars are firm.
Once chilled, lift the bars out of the pan using the parchment paper overhang.
Cut the mixture into bars or squares of your desired size.
Store your No-Bake Peanut Butter and Chocolate Oat Bars in an airtight container in the refrigerator.

Enjoy these delicious and easy-to-make breakfast bars!

<u>Homemade Energy Bites</u>

Ingredients:

1 cup rolled oats
1/2 cup nut butter (e.g., peanut, almond, or cashew butter)
1/3 cup honey or maple syrup
1/2 cup ground flaxseed
1/2 cup mini chocolate chips or dried fruit (e.g., cranberries or apricots)
1/2 cup shredded coconut (optional)
1 teaspoon vanilla extract
A pinch of salt

Instructions:

In a large mixing bowl, combine the rolled oats, ground flaxseed, mini chocolate chips or dried fruit, and shredded coconut (if using).

In a microwave-safe bowl, warm the nut butter and honey (or maple syrup) until they're easy to stir.

This usually takes about 20-30 seconds in the microwave.
Stir the vanilla extract and a pinch of salt into the nut butter and honey mixture.
Pour the nut butter mixture over the dry ingredients in the large mixing bowl.
Mix everything together until well combined.

Chill the mixture in the refrigerator for about 30 minutes.
This will make it easier to handle.

Once chilled, use your hands to roll the mixture into bite-sized balls.

You can make them as small or as large as you prefer.
Place the energy bites on a parchment-lined tray or plate.
Refrigerate the energy bites for another 30 minutes to firm them up.

Transfer the Homemade Energy Bites to an airtight container and store them in the refrigerator.
Enjoy these nutritious and convenient energy-packed bites whenever you need a quick breakfast or snack!

<u>Almond and Cranberry Breakfast Bars</u>

Ingredients:

1 1/2 cups rolled oats
1 cup almond butter
1/2 cup honey or maple syrup
1/2 cup dried cranberries
1/4 cup chopped almonds
1/4 cup ground flaxseed
1 teaspoon vanilla extract
A pinch of salt

Instructions:

In a large mixing bowl, combine the rolled oats, dried cranberries, chopped almonds, and ground flaxseed.
In a microwave-safe bowl, warm the almond butter and honey (or maple syrup) until they're easy to stir.
This usually takes about 20-30 seconds in the microwave.
Stir the vanilla extract and a pinch of salt into the almond butter and honey mixture.
Pour the almond butter mixture over the dry ingredients in the large mixing bowl.
Mix everything together until well combined.
Line an 8x8-inch square baking pan with parchment paper, leaving some overhang on the sides for easy removal.
Press the mixture firmly into the prepared baking pan using a spatula or your hands.
Place the pan in the refrigerator and chill for at least 1-2 hours, or until the bars are firm.
Once chilled, lift the bars out of the pan using the parchment paper overhang.
Cut the mixture into bars or squares of your desired size.
Store your Almond and Cranberry Breakfast Bars in an airtight container in the refrigerator.
Enjoy these wholesome and delicious breakfast bars!

These homemade breakfast bars and bites are convenient, customizable, and perfect for a quick and nutritious morning meal or snack.
Feel free to modify the ingredients to suit your taste preferences.
Enjoy!

Quick & Easy Grab-and-Go Options

<u>Greek Yogurt and Fruit Parfait Cups</u>

Ingredients:

Greek yogurt (plain or flavored)
Mixed berries (strawberries, blueberries, raspberries)
Granola
Honey or maple syrup (optional, for sweetness)

Greek Yogurt and Fruit Parfait Cups are a fantastic choice for a nutritious and convenient breakfast or snack.
Here's why they work so well:
Greek Yogurt: Greek yogurt is rich in protein, which helps keep you full and satisfied. It's also a good source of probiotics, promoting gut health. You can choose plain Greek yogurt or opt for flavored varieties like vanilla or honey for extra flavor.
Mixed Berries: Berries are loaded with vitamins, antioxidants, and fiber. They add a burst of color, flavor, and natural sweetness to your parfait. Plus, they're easy to pack and eat on the go.
Granola: Granola provides a delightful crunch and additional fiber to your parfait. It's often sweetened with honey or maple syrup, adding a touch of sweetness. Be mindful of portion size, as granola can be calorie-dense. Honey or Maple Syrup (optional): If you prefer your parfait a bit sweeter, drizzle some honey or maple syrup over the layers. This is entirely optional and can be adjusted to your taste.

Layer your parfait in a portable container with a lid, such as a mason jar or plastic container, for easy grab-and-go access:
Start with a layer of Greek yogurt at the bottom.
Add a layer of mixed berries.
Sprinkle a layer of granola. If desired, drizzle honey or maple syrup for sweetness.
Repeat the layers until your container is full or until you've reached your desired portion.

These provide a balanced mix of protein, fiber, and vitamins. Easy to prepare ahead of time and store in the fridge for grab-and-go convenience. Customizable with your favorite fruits, nuts, or seeds. Can be a satisfying breakfast or a healthy snack option.

<u>Nut Butter and Banana Rice Cakes:</u>

Ingredients:

Rice cakes
Nut butter (e.g., peanut, almond, or cashew butter)
Bananas

Nut Butter and Banana Rice Cakes are a simple yet satisfying snack or breakfast option, ideal for those hectic mornings or midday cravings.

Here's why they're great:

Rice Cakes: Rice cakes are light, crunchy, and neutral in flavor, making them a versatile base. They're also gluten-free, which accommodates various dietary preferences.

Nut Butter: Nut butter adds healthy fats, protein, and a rich, creamy texture. You can choose your favorite variety, such as peanut, almond, or cashew butter. Nut butter pairs exceptionally well with bananas.

Bananas: Bananas are a quick and convenient fruit choice. They're portable, naturally sweet, and provide essential nutrients like potassium and vitamin C.

Assembling Nut Butter and Banana Rice Cakes is as easy as it gets:
Spread a layer of your preferred nut butter onto each rice cake.
Slice bananas and place them on top of the nut butter.
Sandwich two rice cakes together with banana slices in the middle, creating a compact and portable snack.

Offers a satisfying combination of carbohydrates, healthy fats, and protein.

Provides a quick energy boost.

Suitable for various dietary preferences and allergen considerations.

Portable and mess-free for on-the-go consumption.

<u>Veggie and Hummus Snack Box:</u>

Ingredients:

Sliced vegetables (e.g., carrots, cucumber, bell peppers)
Hummus Cherry tomatoes
Whole-grain crackers (optional)

The Veggie and Hummus Snack Box is a savory, nutrient-packed option for those looking to get their veggies on the go.

Here's why it's a smart choice:

Sliced Vegetables: Colorful vegetables like carrots, cucumber, and bell peppers provide essential vitamins, minerals, and fiber.
They're also hydrating and refreshing.

Hummus: Hummus is a creamy dip made from chickpeas, tahini, and various seasonings.
It offers plant-based protein and healthy fats. The combination of hummus and veggies is both satisfying and nutritious.

Cherry Tomatoes: Cherry tomatoes add a burst of flavor and juiciness to the snack box. They're easy to eat and complement the hummus and veggies.

Whole-Grain Crackers (optional): If you prefer a heartier snack, you can include whole-grain crackers for extra crunch and fiber.

Creating a Veggie and Hummus Snack Box is straightforward:
Place a generous scoop of hummus in a small, portable container with a lid.
Arrange the sliced vegetables and cherry tomatoes in a separate section or container. If including crackers, add them to the box or pack them separately to prevent them from getting soggy.

Provides a balanced combination of protein, fiber, and vitamins.
A savory and satisfying option for those who prefer savory snacks.
Supports hydration due to the water content in vegetables.
Customizable with your favorite veggies and dips.

<u>Trail Mix and Dried Fruit Packets:</u>

Ingredients:

Trail mix (nuts, seeds, dried fruits, and chocolate chips)
Dried fruits (e.g., apricots, raisins, or mango slices)
Portable snack bags or containers

Trail Mix and Dried Fruit Packets are the ultimate grab-and-go snack for active individuals or anyone who needs a quick energy boost.

Here's why: they're a top choice:

Trail Mix: Trail mix typically includes a blend of nuts (e.g., almonds, peanuts), seeds (e.g., sunflower or pumpkin seeds), dried fruits (e.g., cranberries or raisins), and sometimes chocolate chips or M&M's.
It provides a mix of healthy fats, protein, and carbohydrates.

Dried Fruits: Dried fruits are naturally sweet and provide quick energy.
They're a great addition to your snack packet, adding variety and flavor.

Creating Trail Mix and Dried Fruit Packets is incredibly easy:
Fill small, resealable snack bags or portable containers with your desired amount of trail mix.
Add a portion of dried fruits to each bag or container.
You can choose one type of dried fruit or create a mix of your favorites.
Seal the bags or containers securely.
Offers a convenient source of energy for active individuals and those on the go.
Portable and mess-free. Customizable with various nuts, seeds, and dried fruits to suit your taste.
Resealable bags allow for portion control and easy storage.

These quick and easy grab-and-go options cater to various tastes and dietary preferences while ensuring you have a convenient and nutritious choice at your fingertips, whether you're rushing to work, school, or simply need a satisfying snack during the day.

Beverages to Jumpstart Your Day

<u>Energizing Matcha Latte:</u>

Ingredients:

1 teaspoon matcha green tea powder
1 cup hot water (not boiling)
1/2 cup unsweetened almond milk (or your choice of milk)
1 tablespoon honey or maple syrup (optional, for sweetness)

Instructions:

Start by sifting the matcha green tea powder into a bowl to remove any lumps. Heat water to about 175°F (80°C), which is just below boiling.

Too-hot water can make the matcha taste bitter.

Add the hot water to the matcha powder in the bowl.
Use a bamboo whisk or a regular whisk to vigorously whisk the matcha and water together until it forms a smooth and frothy mixture.

This step is crucial for achieving a creamy texture. In a separate saucepan, heat the unsweetened almond milk until it's warm but not boiling.

You can also heat it in the microwave.

If you prefer sweetness, add honey or maple syrup to the milk and stir until it's well combined.

Pour the sweetened almond milk into a mug.
Gently pour the whisked matcha mixture into the almond milk while holding back the froth with a spoon.

You can use a strainer for a smoother texture.
Stir the matcha and almond milk together, ensuring they are well combined.
Your Energizing Matcha Latte is ready to sip and enjoy.

The vibrant green color and earthy flavor make it a delightful and energizing morning drink.

<u>Turmeric Ginger Tea:</u>

Ingredients:

1 cup water
1-inch piece of fresh turmeric (or 1/2 teaspoon ground turmeric)
1-inch piece of fresh ginger
1 teaspoon honey or maple syrup (optional, for sweetness)
A squeeze of fresh lemon juice (optional)

Instructions:

Start by peeling and thinly slicing the fresh turmeric and ginger.

In a saucepan, bring the water to a boil. Add the turmeric and ginger slices to the boiling water.

Reduce the heat to a simmer and let the ingredients steep for about 10-15 minutes.

This allows the flavors to infuse into the water.

If you prefer sweetness, add honey or maple syrup to the tea and stir until it's dissolved.

Remove the saucepan from the heat and strain the turmeric ginger tea into a cup.

If desired, add a squeeze of fresh lemon juice for a bright and zesty flavor.

Your Turmeric Ginger Tea is ready to sip and enjoy.

This aromatic and soothing tea is known for its potential health benefits and is perfect for a warm and comforting start to your day.

Freshly Squeezed Orange Juice:

Ingredients:

4-6 ripe oranges

Instructions:

Begin by washing and scrubbing the oranges thoroughly.
Cut each orange in half.

Using a citrus juicer or a handheld reamer, squeeze the juice from each
orange half into a pitcher or glass.

Make sure to remove any seeds.

If you like, you can chill the orange juice in the refrigerator before serving.

Your Freshly Squeezed Orange Juice is ready to enjoy.

The natural sweetness and vibrant flavor of freshly squeezed orange juice

make it a refreshing and invigorating choice to kickstart your day.

<u>Iced Green Tea with Mint:</u>

Ingredients:

2 green tea bags
2 cups hot water
Fresh mint leaves Honey or maple syrup (optional, for sweetness)
Ice cubes

Instructions:

Place the green tea bags in a heatproof container or teapot.
Pour hot water over the tea bags.
Let the tea steep for about 3-5 minutes, or until it reaches your desired strength.
Remove the tea bags and allow the tea to cool to room temperature.

If you prefer sweetness, add honey or maple syrup to the tea and stir until it's dissolved.

Once the tea is cooled, transfer it to a refrigerator and let it chill for at least 30 minutes.

To serve, fill a glass with ice cubes and pour the chilled green tea over the ice.

Garnish with fresh mint leaves for a burst of flavor and aroma.

Your Iced Green Tea with Mint is ready to enjoy.

This refreshing and antioxidant-rich beverage is perfect for a cool and revitalizing morning pick-me-up.

These beverages offer a variety of flavors and health benefits to help you start your day feeling refreshed and energized.

Enjoy your morning beverages!